The Vegan Bodybuilder's Cookbook

The last 40 vegan recipes for beginners and experienced that help you to grow your muscles, decrease stress, have a healthy mind and an energized body.

Daniel Wilson

Test of Contents

Introduction

The plant-based diet is one of the most efficient ways to lose weight. It is better than another non-vegetarian dieting with vegans giving the best results. It takes a lot of self-discipline and patience to follow the diet, but in the end, all that is rewarded with your goals being achieved.

You need to plan if you are thinking about dieting. First, you can start slowly by just eating one meal a day, which is vegetarian and gradually increasing your number of vegetarian meals. Whenever you are struggling, ask your friend or family member to support you and keep you motivated. One important thing is also to be regularly accountable for not following the diet.

If dieting seems very important to you and you need to do it right, then it is recommended that you visit a professional such as a nutritionist or dietitian to discuss your dieting plan and optimizing it for the better.

No matter how much you want to lose weight, it is not advised that you decrease your calorie intake to an unhealthy level. Losing weight does not mean that you stop eating. It is done by carefully planning meals.

A plant-based diet is very easy once you get into it. At first, you will start to face a lot of difficulties, but if you start slowly, then you can face all the barriers and achieve your goal.

Healthy plant-derived protein tends to be high in vitamins, minerals, fiber, antioxidants and various other substances that we require to remain healthy and balanced. Some kinds include considerable quantities of healthy and balanced fats, as well. Beans, nuts, seeds and entire groups of grains are all healthy plant proteins that you should consume.

Research studies have revealed that healthy plant protein, as part of a plant-based diet plan, lowered the body weight and enhanced insulin resistance in obese individuals. If you are looking to reach your healthy and balanced weight, including even more plants to your diet plan is a terrific step, to begin with.

The next step is to decide how and when you are going to make the switch. Whether you choose to do it slowly, or you prefer to jump right in, the important thing is that you have made the decision. Within a short time, you should notice many positive changes and improvements in how your body feels and responds during periods of physical activity. You should see how much better you are able to train and compete as well as feel much better overall.

At first, it may take a little bit of getting used to, once you have switched to the fully vegan diet. Though, it will not take long for your body to eliminate all of the "bad stuff". Once this happens, you should notice that you have made the right decision, not only for your health, but also to improve your sports performance.

Start making changes in your diet. It's in your hands now. You have the facts about veganism and bodybuilding, and now it is up to you to decide how you are going to make the switch. It's a big switch to make, too, but it is completely doable. I like to suggest that you start with eating vegan two to three times a week and eat the way you are used to the rest of the week, for a month or so. This can help you get familiarize to your new diet and will help your body to adjust.

Appetizer and
Snack Recipes

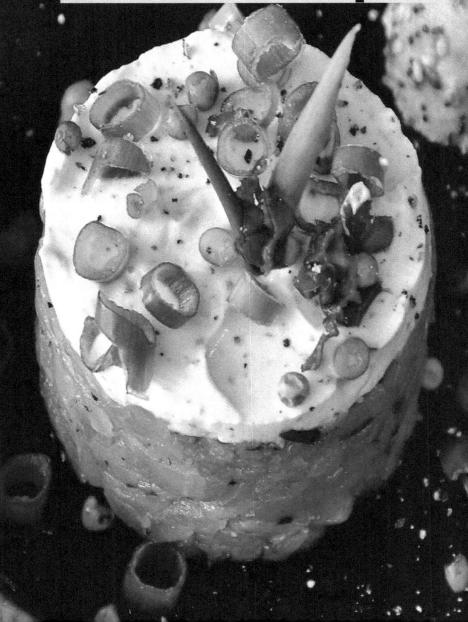

1. Sunflower Seed Bites

Preparation Time: 10 minutes

Cooking Time: 0 minute

Servings: 4

Ingredients

- ¾ cup of sunflower seeds
- ½ cup of dates (pitted)
- 3 tbsp of raw cacao
- 2 tbsp of agave
- 1 tbsp of coconut oil
- ½ tsp of cinnamon
- ¼ tsp of nutmeg
- ¼ tsp of Himalayan salt

Direction

1.   Add the sunflower seeds to a blender and blend it on medium-high speed until it is a fine meal consistency. Don't over-blend the sunflower seeds, as it will turn into butter.

2.   Add the raw cacao, dates, coconut oil, agave, cinnamon, nutmeg, and Himalayan salt until you've reached a dough consistency.

3.   Form the dough by rolling it into 2 ½ to 3-inch balls. Once done, place all the bites on a board, and refrigerate it for 30 minutes.

Nutrition

48 Calories

2g Carbohydrates

1.1g Protein

2.Sweet Nut Bars

Preparation Time: 5 minutes

Cooking Time: 15 minutes

Servings: 4

Ingredients

- 1 ½ cups of mixed raw nuts
- 1 cup of coconut flakes
- ½ cup of hemp seeds
- ½ cup of pumpkin seeds
- ½ cup of sesame seeds
- ½ cup of cranberries
- ½ cup of almond butter
- 4 tbsp of agave
- 1 tsp of cinnamon
- 1 tsp of vanilla extract

Direction

1. Preheat the oven to 350 degrees-Fahrenheit.

2. Line an oven tin with parchment paper.

3. Mix coconut flakes, nuts, cranberries, sesame seeds, hemp seeds, cinnamon, and pumpkin seeds in a bowl to combine.

4. Add the almond butter and agave to the bowl, and mix well. Then, add the vanilla extract and stir once more.

5. Add the bowl mixture to a non-stick pan, and stir everything until well combined.

6. Transfer the mixture to the oven tin, and press it to form an even layer.

7. Bake the bars for 15 minutes before removing it from the oven to cool down.

8. Once cooled, cut it into 10 to 12 bars.

Nutrition

340 Calories

19g Carbohydrates

10.2g Protein

3. Peanut Butter Crunch Rice Cakes

Preparation Time: 5 minutes

Cooking Time: 0 minute

Servings: 4

Ingredients

- 8 medium rice cakes (gluten-free)
- 5 to 6 tbsp of crunchy peanut butter (natural)
- ½ cup of raisins
- ¼ cup of agave

Direction

1. Plate 2 rice cakes per serving, and spread ½ to 1 tbsp of crunchy peanut butter evenly on top.

2. Add some raisins, and a drizzle of agave (optional).

3. Place the 3 to 4 ingredients in small separate containers, and prep per serving.

Nutrition

265 Calories

2.6g Carbohydrates

7g Protein

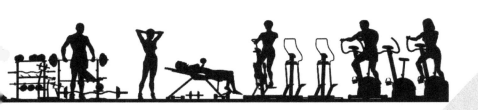

4.Spicy Edamame

Preparation Time: 5 minutes

Cooking Time: 0 minute

Servings: 4

Ingredients

- 2 cups of edamame
- ½ tsp. of Aleppo pepper
- ¼ tsp of black pepper

Direction

1.   Steam the edamame according to its package instructions, remove, and allow it to cool down. Transfer to a bowl.

2.   Sprinkle Aleppo pepper and black pepper on top, and shake the bowl for the spice to cover all the edamame.

Nutrition

100 Calories

9.3g Carbohydrates

8g Protein

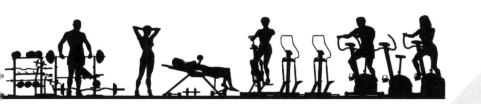

5.Sweet Pistachio Bites

Preparation Time: 10 minutes

Cooking Time: 0 minute

Servings: 4

Ingredients

- 2 cups of dates
- 1 cup of cranberries
- 1 cup of pistachios
- 1 tsp of pumpkin seeds
- ¼ tsp of black pepper

Direction

1.　　Blend dates, cranberries, pistachios, pumpkin seeds, and black pepper to a high-performance food processor.

2.　　Roll the date dough into 2 ½ to 3-inch round balls, usually 1 tbsp each.

Nutrition

70 Calories

13.2g Carbohydrates

1.2g Protein

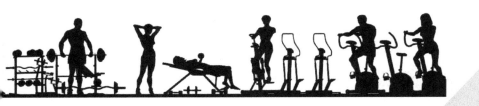

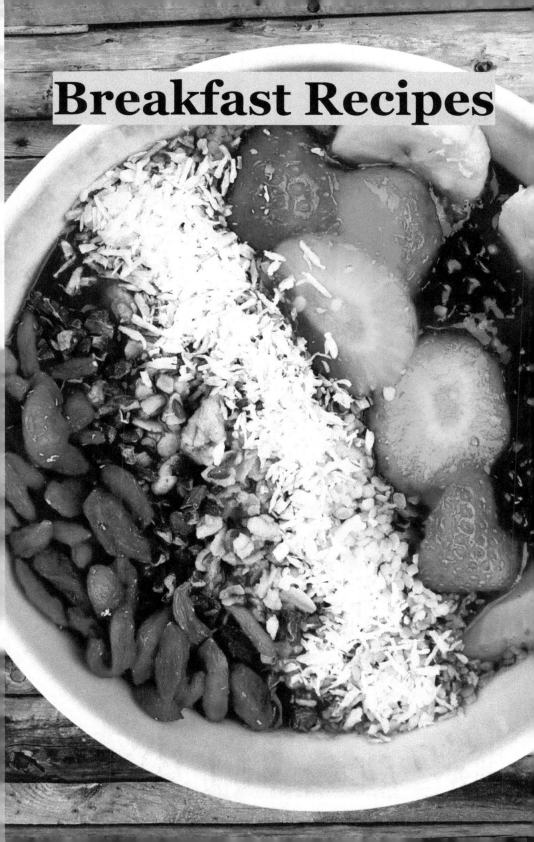

Breakfast Recipes

6.No-Bake Vegan Protein Bar

Preparation Time: 20 minutes

Cooking Time: 0 minute

Serving: 5

Ingredients:

- 1/3 cup amaranth
- 3 tbsp. vanilla vegan protein powder.
- 2 tbsp maple syrup.
- 1 cup almond butter.
- 3 tbsp. dark vegan chocolate.

Direction:

1. In 8 x 8-inch baking pan, place parchment paper and set aside.
2. Pop your amaranth by heating a big pot over medium-high heat.
3. Include about 2-3 tbsp amaranth at a time and right away cover. Shake over the heat to move the grain around.

4. Not every single grain will pop.
5. Do not blend any scorched grain with the completely popped grain. Set aside.
6. Mix in almond butter and maple syrup. Then add protein powder and stir.
7. Include popped amaranth a little at a time until you have a loose "dough" texture.
8. Transfer the mixture to the baking meal and press down to form an even layer. Lay parchment paper or plastic wrap on the top.
9. Transfer to freezer to set for 10-15 minutes or until firm to the touch. Lift out and slice it into nine bars.

Nutrition:

215 Calories

15g Fat

10.7g Protein

7. Orange Pumpkin Pancakes

Preparation Time: 15 minutes

Cooking Time: 10 minutes

Serving: 4

Ingredients:

- 10 g ground flax meal
- 45 ml water
- 235 ml unsweetened soy milk
- 15 ml lemon juice
- 60 g buckwheat flour
- 60 g all-purpose flour
- 8 g baking powder
- 2 tsp finely grated orange zest
- 25 g white chia seeds
- 120 g organic pumpkin puree
- 30 ml melted and cooled coconut oil
- 5 ml vanilla paste
- 30 ml pure maple syrup

Direction

1. Combine ground flax meal with water. Place aside for 10 minutes. Combine almond milk and cider vinegar. Place aside for 5 minutes.
2. Mix buckwheat flour, all-purpose flour, baking powder, orange zest, and chia seeds.
3. Whisk almond milk, along with pumpkin puree, coconut oil, vanilla, and maple syrup.
4. Heat large non-stick skillet over medium-high heat. Brush the skillet gently with some coconut oil.
5. Pour 60ml of batter into skillet. Cook the pancake for 1 minute. Flip.
6. Cook 1 1/2 minutes more. Slide the pancake onto a plate. Repeat with the remaining batter.

Nutrition:

301 Calories

12.6g fat

8.1g Protein

8. Sweet Potato Slices with Fruits

Preparation Time: 15 minutes

Cooking Time: 10 minutes

Serving: 2

Ingredients:

- 1 sweet potato

Topping.

- 60 g organic peanut butter.
- 30ml pure maple syrup.
- 4 dried apricots, sliced.
- 30 g fresh raspberries.

Direction

1. Peel and slice sweet potato into 1/2 cm thick slices.
2. Place the potato slices in a toaster on high for 5 minutes. Toast your sweet potatoes TWICE.
3. Arrange sweet potato slices onto a plate.

4. Spread the peanut butter over sweet potato slices.

5. Drizzle the maple syrup over the butter. Top each slice with an equal amount of sliced apricots and raspberries. Serve.

Nutrition:

300 Calories

16.9g fat

10.3g Protein

9.Pumpkin Sourdough Protein Pancakes

Preparation Time: 30 minutes

Cooking Time: 5 minutes

Serving: 5

Overnight sponge:

- 1/4 cup gluten-free sourdough starter.
- 1/4 cup pumpkin puree.
- 1/2 cup chickpea flour
- 1/2 cup almond milk.
- 1-2 tbsp. maple syrup.

In the morning:

- 1 flax egg
- 1 tsp. pumpkin spice.
- 1 tsp. cinnamon.
- 1/2 tsp. turmeric.
- 1/4 cup raw cacao nibs
- A handful of sliced pecans

- 1/2 tsp. baking soda.
- 1 tsp. baking powder.

Direction:

1. The night before making the pancakes, position the overnight sponge ingredients into a non-reactive bowl. Mix well, cover with plastic wrap.
2. In the morning, before making pancakes, mix all the other ingredients (except baking powder and baking soda) into the overnight sponge.
3. Heat a non-stick pan over medium heat.
4. Stir in baking soda and baking powder to the batter and carefully stir them in.
5. Put 1/4 cup of the batter onto the pan for each pancake and fry until you see bubbles forming on the surface area of the pancakes and the edges dry out.

Nutrition:

543 Calories

1.1g Fat

4.3g Protein

10. Energizing Daily Tonic

Preparation Time: 15 minutes

Cooking Time: 0 minute

Serving: 2

Ingredients base:

- 2-4 tbsp. vegan protein powder.
- 1 tbsp. maca powder.
- 1 tsp. ashwagandha powder.
- 1 tsp. mushroom blend powder.
- 1 tsp. astragalus powder.
- 1/4 cup pecans.
- 2 Brazil nuts.
- Pinch of stevia powder.
- 1-2 tbsp. maple syrup or dates

Add-ons:

- 1 tbsp. cacao powder.
- 1 tbsp. ground coffee.
- 1/2 tsp. vanilla extract.

Direction

1. Blend all the base active ingredients except the maple syrup up until smooth, velvety and tasty. Include 1 to 2 tablespoons of maple syrup or a small handful of dates, if you desire it sweeter.
2. Sprinkle with apple pie spice, if utilizing, and enjoy!

Nutrition

160 Calories

5.5g Protein

0.8g fat

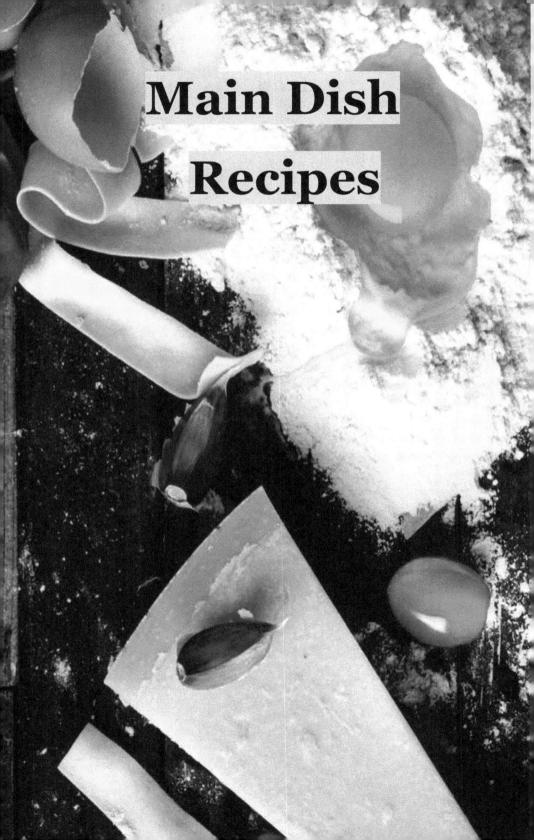

Main Dish Recipes

11. Iron Abs Tabbouleh

Preparation Time: 15 minutes

Cooking Time: 10 minutes

Serving: 4

Ingredients

- 1 cup whole-wheat couscous
- 1 cup boiling water
- Zest and juice of 1 lemon
- 1 garlic clove, pressed
- Pinch of sea salt
- 1 tablespoon olive oil
- 2 cups canned chickpeas
- ½ cucumber
- 1 tomato
- 1 cup fresh parsley
- ¼ cup fresh mint
- 2 scallions
- 4 tablespoons sunflower seeds

Direction

1. Soak couscous with boiling water until all the grains are submerged. Cover. Set aside.
2. Put the lemon zest and juice in a large salad bowl, then stir in the garlic, salt, and the olive oil
3. Put the cucumber, chickpeas, tomato, parsley, mint, and scallions in the bowl, and toss them to coat with the dressing. Stir with fork
4. Stir in cooked couscous to the vegetables, and toss to combine.
5. Serve topped with the sunflower seeds

Nutrition

304 Calories

11g fat

10g Protein

12. Mushroom Cream

Preparation Time: 10 minutes

Cooking Time: 20 minutes

Serving: 2

Ingredients

- 2 teaspoons olive oil
- 1 onion
- 2 garlic cloves
- 2 cups chopped mushrooms
- 2 tablespoons whole-grain flour
- 1 teaspoon dried herbs
- 4 cups Economical Vegetable Broth
- 1½ cups nondairy milk

Direction

1. Preheat oil over medium-high heat.
2. Add the onion, garlic, mushrooms, and salt. Sauté for about 5 minutes, until softened. Throw flour over the ingredients in the pot and mix.
3. Cook for 1 to 2 minutes more to toast the flour.

4. Add the dried herbs, vegetable broth, milk, and pepper.
5. Set heat to low, and let the broth come to a simmer.
6. Cook for 10 minutes, until slightly thickened.

Nutrition:

127 Calories

10g Protein

3g Fiber

13. Fast Twitch Quinoa

Preparation Time: 5 minutes

Cooking Time: 0 minute

Serving: 7

Ingredients

- 3 tablespoons olive oil
- Juice of 1½ lemons
- 1 teaspoon garlic powder
- ½ teaspoon dried oregano
- 1 bunch curly kale
- 2 cups cooked tricolor quinoa
- 1 cup canned mandarin oranges in juice
- 1 cup diced yellow summer squash
- 1 red bell pepper
- ½ red onion
- ½ cup dried cranberries
- ½ cup slivered almonds

Direction

1. Scourge the oil, lemon juice, garlic powder, and oregano.
2. Mix the kale with the oil-lemon mixture until well coated. Add the quinoa, oranges, squash, bell pepper, and red onion and toss until all the ingredients are well combined. Divide among bowls or transfer to a large serving platter. Top with the cranberries and almonds.

Nutrition:

343 Calories

24g Protein

11g Fiber

14. Eggplant Parmesan

Preparation Time: 10 minutes

Cooking Time: 15 minutes

Serving: 1

Ingredients

- ¼ cup nondairy milk
- ¼ cup bread crumbs or panko
- 2 tablespoons nutritional yeast
- ¼ teaspoon salt
- 4 (¼-inch-thick) eggplant slices
- 1 tablespoon olive oil
- 4 tablespoons Simple Homemade Tomato Sauce
- 4 teaspoons Pram Sprinkle

Direction

1. Put the milk in a shallow bowl. Blend the bread crumbs, nutritional yeast and salt.
2. Dip one eggplant slice in the milk, making sure both sides get moistened. Dip it into the bread crumbs, flipping to coat both sides. Transfer to a plate and repeat

to coat the remaining slices. Preheat oil over medium heat and add the breaded eggplant slices.

3. Cook for 6 minutes. Flip, adding more oil as needed. Top each slice with 1 tablespoon tomato sauce and 1 teaspoon Pram Sprinkle. Cook for 5 to 7 minutes more.

Nutrition:

460 Calories

9g Protein

13g Fiber

15. Pepper & Kale

Preparation Time: 5 minutes

Cooking Time: 15 minutes

Serving: 4

Ingredients

- 2 cans chickpeas
- 4 cloves garlic
- 1 large sweet onion
- 4 tbsp olive oil
- 2 red peppers
- 6 cups kale

Direction

1. Heat BBQ and prepare a greased BBQ basket or pan.
2. Meanwhile, mix together chickpeas, garlic, onion, red peppers and olive oil in a bowl and add to the BBQ basket and place on the grill. Stir regularly.
3. When almost ready to serve add kale and stir constantly until the kale is slightly wilted. Serve with garlic toast, pita bread or rice.

Nutrition:

520 Calories

16g Fiber

18g Protein

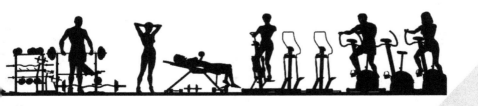

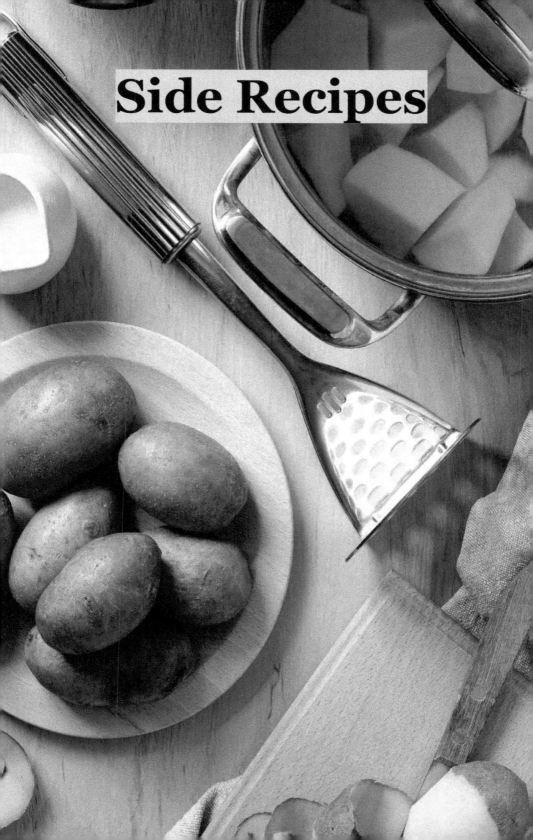

Side Recipes

16. Buffalo Chickpeas and Lettuce Wraps

Preparation Time: 10 minutes

Cooking Time: 5 minutes

Serving: 2

Ingredients

- Olive oil - 1 tablespoon
- Chickpeas - 1 can (15 ounces)
- Garlic powder - ½ teaspoon
- Salt - 1 pinch
- Buffalo sauce - ¼ cup
- Hummus – 1/3 cup
- Lemon juice - 1 tablespoon
- Water - 1 tablespoon
- Tortillas - 2 large
- Romaine lettuce – 4 leaves
- Red onion (sliced)
- Tomato (sliced)

Directions

1.Take a large nonstick saucepan and pour 1 tablespoon of olive oil. Place it over medium flame.

2.Once the oil starts simmering, toss in the chickpeas and cook for about 3 minutes.

3. Add in the salt, buffalo sauce and garlic powder. Cook for about 2 minutes. Coat the chickpeas well. Keep aside.

4.Mix hummus, water and lemon juice.

5.Now take the tortillas and place 2 romaine lettuce leaves in the center. Top it with chickpeas, sliced tomatoes and sliced red onions.

6.Pour the hummus dressing on top.

7.Fold the edges and roll it in the shape of a burrito. Cut in equal halves.

8.Repeat the process with the other tortilla.

Nutrition

19g Fat

89g Carbohydrates

25g Protein

17. Lentil and Cheese Nuggets

Preparation Time: 10 minutes

Cooking Time: 20 minutes

Serving: 6

Ingredients

- Lentils - 1 ½ cups
- Carrot (sliced) - 1
- Corn - ½ cup
- Pea - ½ cup
- Vegan cheddar cheese (shredded) - 1 cup
- Dried oregano - 1 teaspoon
- Salt - 1 teaspoon
- Pepper - 1 teaspoon
- Red pepper flakes - ½ teaspoon
- Garlic - 1 clove

Directions

1. Start by soaking the lentil for 3 hours in cold water.

2. Once the lentils are done soaking, set the temperature of the oven at 400 degrees Fahrenheit and let it preheat.

3. In a baking tray and line it using parchment paper.

4. Now take a food processor and add in the carrots, peas, corns, vegan cheddar cheese, salt, oregano, pepper, garlic, soaked lentils and red pepper flakes. Pulse to mix all the ingredients well.

5. Form nuggets by taking 1 tablespoon of lentil mixture using your hands. Repeat the process with the rest of the mixture.

6. Place all the nuggets onto the lined baking tray. Bake for about 10 minutes. Turnover and bake again for 10 minutes.

7. Remove the baking tray from the oven and let the cutlets rest for about 5 minutes. Serve!

Nutrition

7g Fat

24g Carbohydrates

13g Protein

18. Black Bean and Sweet Potato Burritos

Preparation Time: 10 minutes

Cooking Time: 30 minutes

Serving: 3

Ingredients

- Sweet potatoes (peel and cut in cubes) - 2
- Smoked paprika - ½ teaspoon
- Garlic powder - ½ teaspoon
- Kosher salt – as per taste
- Pepper – as per taste
- Yellow onion (diced) - ½ medium
- Jalapeño (diced) - ½ medium
- Garlic (minced) - 1 clove
- Chili powder - 1 teaspoon
- Ground cumin - ½ teaspoon
- Cayenne pepper – as per taste
- Black beans (drain and rinse) - 1 can
- Corn - ¾ cup
- Flour tortillas - 3 large

Directions

1. Start by preheating the oven by setting the temperature to 400 degrees Fahrenheit.

2. Take a nonstick baking tray and toss in the cubed sweet potatoes. Drizzle olive oil on top. Also sprinkle the garlic powder, paprika, pepper and salt. Toss well to ensure the sweet potatoes are evenly coated.

3. Place the tray in the preheated oven and bake for about 10 minutes. Turn over the sweet potatoes and bake again for 10 minutes.

4. Take a nonstick saucepan and drizzle olive oil. Place it over medium flame.

5. Once the oil starts simmering, toss in the onions and cook for about 4 minutes.

6. Add in the garlic, jalapeno, cumin, cayenne pepper and chili powder. Cook for another 3 minutes.

7. Toss in the black beans, pepper and salt and cook for 3 minutes. The ingredients should completely heat through.

8. Let us now assemble the burrito, place one of the tortillas on a flat surface. Add 1/3 of corn and bean mixture, 1/3 of prepared sweet potatoes, little bit of lettuce, guacamole, diced tomatoes and vegan cheddar

cheese in the center. Crease the edges and roll to form a burrito. Repeat the process the remaining tortillas.

9. Cut each burrito in two equal halves and serve.

Nutrition

12g Fat

95g Carbohydrates

16g Protein

19. Mac and Peas and Cashew Sauce

Preparation Time: 10 minutes

Cooking Time: 10 minutes

Serving: 4

Ingredients

- Yellow potatoes - 2
- Carrot) - 1 medium
- Onion) - 1
- Cashews - ½ cup
- Salt - 1 teaspoon
- Garlic powder - 1 teaspoon
- Onion powder - 1 teaspoon
- Nutritional yeast - 2 tablespoons
- Macaroni (cooked) - 16 ounces
- Green peas - 2 cups

Directions

1. Start by taking a large pot with water and place it over high heat. When it comes to a boil add in the carrots, onions and potatoes. Cover and boil for t 10 minutes.

2. Remove the boiled vegetables using a strainer. Reserve about 2 cups of water for later use.

3. Take a blender and add in the boiled carrots, onions, potatoes, cashews, salt, garlic powder, onion powder, nutritional yeast, paprika along with the reserved water. Blend well to form smooth puree like consistency.

4. Toss cooked macaroni and puree on top. Then green peas and mix well. Serve!

Nutrition

7g Fat

105g Carbohydrates

21g Protein

20. Baked Deep-Dish Apple Pancake

Preparation time: 10 minutes

Cooking Time: 35 minutes

Serving: 6

Ingredients

- 4 tart apples
- ¼ cup (30 g) chopped walnuts
- 1 teaspoon ground cinnamon
- 1½ cups (225 g) whole wheat flour
- 2 teaspoons baking powder
- ¼ teaspoon plus 1/8 teaspoon salt
- 1 cup (240 ml) light or full-fat coconut milk
- 2 tablespoons maple syrup
- 1 tablespoon lemon juice
- 1 teaspoon vanilla extract
- ¼ cup coconut sugar
- 1 tablespoon coconut oil

Direction:

1. Preheat the oven at 190 ° C. Place on medium heat a deep cast-iron skillet. Once warm, add in a single layer the apples, ½ teaspoon cinnamon, and walnuts if used. Let the apples cook while the batter is being cooked.
2. Mix the flour, baking powder, ¼ teaspoon salt, and ½ teaspoon cinnamon remaining. Stir the coconut milk, maple syrup, 1 tablespoon of lemon juice and vanilla then pour into the dry ingredients and whisk until mixed.
3. Sprinkle the sugar, 1 teaspoon of lemon juice left over the apples, and 1/8 teaspoon of salt. Remove from the heat, apply the coconut oil to the pan, concentrating on the apples ' perimeter.
4. Spoon the batter over the top and bake for 30 to 35 minutes. Slice into wedges, pick and serve on bowls.

Nutrition

17g Fat

103g Carbohydrates

83g Protein

Vegetable Recipes

21. Green Beans Gremolata

Preparation Time: 15 minutes

Cooking Time: 5 minutes

Serving: 6

Ingredients:

- 1-pound fresh green beans
- 3 garlic cloves, minced
- Zest of 2 oranges
- 3 tablespoons minced fresh parsley
- 2 tablespoons pine nuts
- 3 tablespoons olive oil
- Sea salt
- Freshly ground black pepper

Direction:

1. Boil water over high heat. Cook green beans for 3 minutes. Drain r and rinse with cold water to stop the cooking.

2. Blend garlic, orange zest, and parsley.

3. In a huge sauté pan over medium-high heat, toast the pine nuts in the dry, hot pan for 3 minutes. Remove from the pan and set aside.

4. Cook olive oil in the same pan until it shimmers. Add the beans and cook, -stirring frequently, until heated through, about 2 minutes. Take pan away from the heat and add the parsley mixture and pine nuts. Season with salt and pepper. Serve immediately.

Nutrition:

98 Calories

2g Fiber

3g Protein

22. Minted Peas

Preparation Time: 5 minutes

Cooking Time: 5 minutes

Serving: 4

Ingredient:

- 1 tablespoon olive oil
- 4 cups peas, fresh or frozen (not canned)
- ½ teaspoon sea salt
- Freshly ground black pepper
- 3 tablespoons chopped fresh mint

Direction:

1. In a large sauté pan, cook olive oil over medium-high heat until hot. Add the peas and cook, about 5 minutes. Remove the pan from heat. Stir in the salt, season with pepper, and stir in the mint. Serve hot.

Nutrition:

90 Calories

5g Fiber

8g Protein

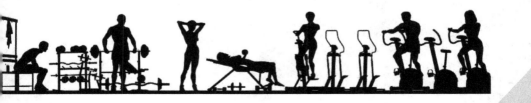

23. Sweet and Spicy Brussels Sprout Hash

Preparation Time: 10 minutes

Cooking Time: 15 minutes

Serving: 4

Ingredient:

- 3 tablespoons olive oil
- 2 shallots, thinly sliced
- 1½ pounds Brussel sprouts
- 3 tablespoons apple cider vinegar
- 1 tablespoon pure maple syrup
- ½ teaspoon sriracha sauce (or to taste)
- Sea salt
- Freshly ground black pepper

Direction

1. In pan, cook olive oil over medium-high heat until it shimmers. Mix the shallots and Brussels sprouts and cook, stirring frequently, until the -vegetables soften and begin to turn golden brown, about 10 minutes. Stir in the

vinegar, using a spoon to scrape any browned bits from the bottom of the pan. Stir in the maple syrup and Sriracha.

2. Simmer, stirring frequently, until the liquid reduces, 3 to 5 minutes. Season and serve immediately.

Nutrition:

97 Calories

4g Fiber

7g Protein

24. Glazed Curried Carrots

Preparation Time: 5 minutes

Cooking Time: 15 minutes

Serving: 6

Ingredient:

- 1-pound carrots
- 2 tablespoons olive oil
- 2 tablespoons curry powder
- 2 tablespoons pure maple syrup
- Juice of ½ lemon

Direction

1. Cook carrots with water over medium-high heat for 10 minutes. Drain and return them to the pan over medium-low heat.
2. Stir in the olive oil, curry powder, maple syrup, and lemon juice. Cook, stirring constantly, until the liquid reduces, about 5 minutes. Season well and serve immediately.

Nutrition:

91 Calories

5g Fiber

9g Protein

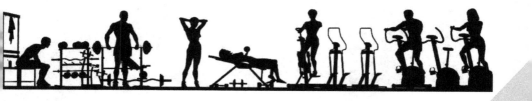

25. Pepper Medley

Preparation Time: 10 minutes

Cooking Time: 15 minutes

Serving: 4

Ingredient:

- 3 tablespoons olive oil
- 1 red bell pepper, sliced
- 1 orange bell pepper, sliced
- 1 yellow bell pepper, sliced
- 1 green bell pepper, sliced
- 2 garlic cloves, minced
- 3 tablespoons red wine vinegar
- 2 tablespoons chopped fresh basil

Direction:

1. Warm up olive oil over medium-high heat. Stir in the bell peppers and cook, stir, for 7 to 10 minutes. Cook garlic for 30 seconds. Add the vinegar, using a spoon to scrape any browned bits off the bottom of the pan.
2. Simmer until the vinegar reduces, 2 to 3 minutes. Season. Stir in the basil and serve immediately.

Nutrition:

96 Calories

3g Fiber

5g Protein

Soup and Stew Recipes

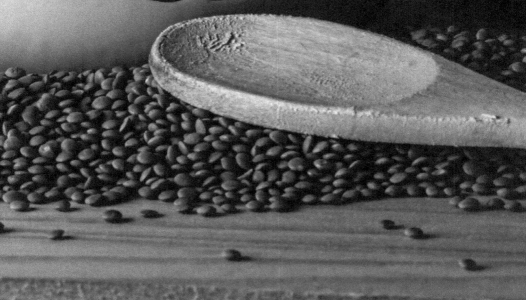

26. Red Lentil Soup

Preparation Time: 10 minutes

Cooking Time: 55 minutes

Serving: 4

Ingredients:

- 1 tbsp. of peanut oil
- 1 small onion, chopped
- 1 tbsp. of minced fresh ginger root
- 1 clove garlic, chopped
- 1 pinch fenugreek seeds
- 1 c. red lentils
- 1 c. of butternut squash
- 1/3 c. fresh cilantro
- 2 c. of water
- ½ (14 oz.) can coconut milk
- 2 tbsp. of tomato paste
- 1 tsp. of curry powder
- 1 pinch cayenne pepper
- 1 pinch ground nutmeg

Direction:

1.   Cook oil in a huge pot over medium heat.

2.   Sauté onion, ginger, garlic, and fenugreek.

3.   Combine the lentils, squash, and cilantro into the pot.

4.   Blend the water, coconut milk, and tomato paste.

5.   Sprinkle curry powder, cayenne pepper, nutmeg, salt, and pepper.

6.   Boil, lower heat, then simmer for about 30 minutes, or until lentils and squash are tender.

7.   Enjoy!

Nutrition:

303 Calories

13g Protein

15g Fat

27. Vegan Chili

Preparation Time: 10 minutes

Cooking Time: 40 minutes

Serving: 5

Ingredients:

- 1 (12 oz.) package vegetarian burger crumbles
- 1 (15 oz.) can tomato sauce
- 1 c. of water
- 1 small onion, chopped
- 3 cloves garlic, minced
- 1 tbsp. of vegetarian Worcestershire sauce
- 1 tsp. of liquid smoke flavoring
- 2 tsp. of chili powder
- 1/8 tsp. of black pepper
- 1 tsp. of dry mustard
- 1 tsp. of salt
- 1/8 tsp. of red pepper flakes

Direction:

1. Mix crumbles, tomato sauce, water, onion, garlic, Worcestershire sauce, liquid smoke, chili powder, black pepper, mustard, salt and pepper flakes.

2. Cook on low heat for 30 minutes.

Nutrition:

147 Calories

15g Protein

4g Fat

28. Vegan Black Bean Soup

Preparation Time: 10 minutes

Cooking Time: 45 minutes

Serving: 6

Ingredients:

- 1 tbsp. of olive oil
- 1 large onion, chopped
- 1 stalk celery, chopped
- 2 medium carrots, chopped
- 4 cloves garlic, chopped
- 2 tbsp. of chili powder
- 1 tbsp. of ground cumin
- 1 pinch black pepper
- 4 c. of vegetable broth
- 4 (15 oz.) cans black beans
- 1 (15 oz.) can whole kernel corn
- 1 (15 oz.) can crushed tomatoes

Direction:

1. Cook oil in a huge pot over medium-high heat.

2. Sauté onion, celery, carrots and garlic for about 5 minutes.

3. Sprinkle with chili powder, cumin, and black pepper; cook for a minute.

4. Boil vegetable broth, 2 cans of beans, and corn.

5. In a food processor or blender, process remaining 2 cans beans and tomatoes until smooth.

6. Stir into boiling soup mixture, reduce heat to medium, and simmer for about 15 minutes.

Nutrition:

410 Calories

22g Protein

5g Fat

29. Vegan Hot and Sour Soup

Preparation Time: 5 minutes

Cooking Time: 1 hour

Serving: 4

Ingredients:

- 1 oz. of dried wood ear mushrooms
- 4 mushrooms dried shiitake mushrooms
- 12 dried tiger lily buds
- 2 c. of hot water
- 1/3 oz. of bamboo fungus
- 3 tbsp. of soy sauce
- 5 tbsp. of rice vinegar
- ¼ c. of cornstarch
- 1 (8 oz. container firm tofu
- 1-quart vegetable broth
- ¼ tsp. of crushed red pepper flakes
- ½ tsp. of ground black pepper
- ¾ tsp. of ground white pepper
- ½ tbsp. of chili oil
- ½ tbsp. of sesame oil

- 1 green onion, sliced
- 1 c. of Chinese dried mushrooms

Direction:

1.   Soak wood mushrooms, shiitake mushrooms, and lily buds in 1 ½ c. of hot water for 20 minutes.

2.   Drain, reserving liquid.

3.   Trim stems from the mushrooms, and slice into thin strips.

4.   Cut the lily buds in half.

5.   Soak bamboo fungus in ¼ c. of lightly salted hot water, in a separate small bowl.

6.   Soak for about 20 minutes, until rehydrated. Drain, and mince.

7.   In a third tiny bowl, mix soy sauce, rice vinegar, and 1 tbsp. of cornstarch.

8.   Place ½ the tofu strips into the mixture.

9.   Combine the reserved mushroom and lily bud liquid with the vegetable broth in a medium saucepan.

10.   Boil wood mushrooms, shiitake mushrooms, and lily buds. Reduce heat, and simmer for 4 minutes.

11.   Sprinkle with red pepper, black pepper, and white pepper.

12.   Combine remaining cornstarch and remaining water in a small bowl.

13.   Stir into the broth mixture until thickened.

14.   Combine soy sauce mix and remaining tofu strips into the saucepan. Return to boil, and mix in the bamboo fungus, chili oil, and sesame oil.

15.   Garnish with green onion to serve.

Nutrition:

238 Calories

13g Protein

9g Fat

30. Sweet Potato Minestrone

Preparation Time: 10 minutes

Cooking Time: 1 hour

Servings: 6

Ingredients:

- 1 tbsp. of vegetable oil
- 1 large onion, chopped
- 2 large stalks celery, chopped
- 2 ½ tsp. of Italian seasoning
- salt and pepper to taste
- 1 (28 oz.) can Italian-style diced tomatoes
- 5 c. of vegetable broth
- 2 large sweet potatoes, peeled and diced
- 2 large carrots, sliced thin
- 6 oz. green beans
- 5 cloves garlic, minced

Direction:

1.   Cook oil in a soup pot over medium-high heat.

2.   Sauté onion, celery, Italian seasoning, salt and pepper until tender, for about 5 minutes.

3.   Mix in tomatoes, with the juice, broth, sweet potatoes, carrots, green beans and garlic.

4.   Boil; decrease the heat then simmer for 30 minutes.

Nutrition:

201 Calories

5g Protein

3g Fat

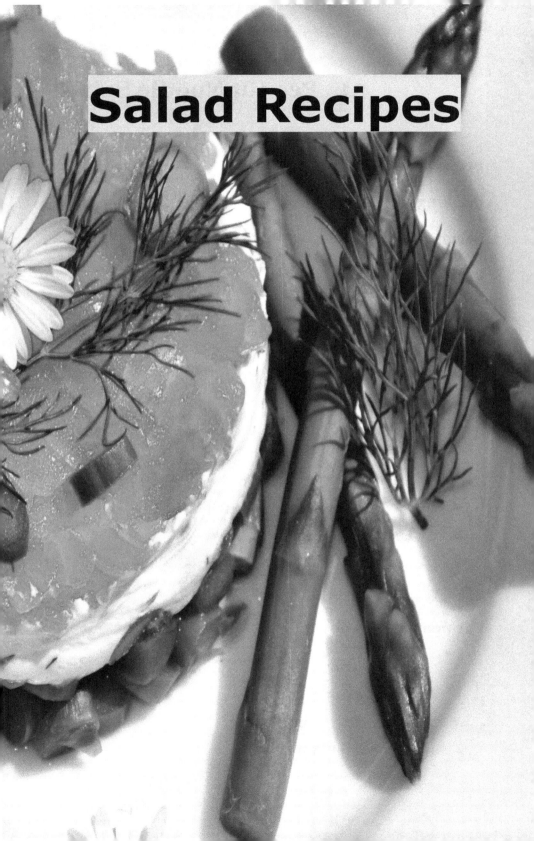

Salad Recipes

31. Peanut Noodle Salad

Preparation Time: 20 minutes

Cooking Time: 5 minutes

Serving: 2

Ingredients:

For salad:

- 1 cup Carrots, shredded
- 1/3 cup Peanuts, chopped
- 8 oz. Rice Noodles
- ½ of 1 Red Bell Pepper, sliced thinly
- 2 Scallions, chopped
- ½ tsp. Black Sesame Seeds

For peanut dressing:

- 3 tbsp. Sriracha
- 2 tbsp. Hot Water
- 2 Garlic cloves, minced
- 1/3 cup Peanut Butter, creamy

- 1 tbsp. Rice Vinegar

Direction:

1. First, cook the noodles by following the instructions given on the packet.
2. Drain the excess water and then rinse it under cold water. Keep aside.
3. After that, combine all the ingredients needed to make the dressing in a small bowl until mixed well. Set it aside.
4. Mix the noodles with all the remaining ingredients and dressing.
5. Combine and then place in the refrigerator until you're ready to serve.

Nutrition:

604 Calories

25g Protein

90g Carbohydrates

32. Broccoli Edamame Salad

Preparation Time: 10 minutes

Cooking Time: 20 minutes

Serving: 5

Ingredients:

For salad:

- 1 Broccoli head, large & torn into florets
- 1 cup Edamame, shelled & cooked
- ½ cup Peanuts
- Sesame Seeds, as needed, for garnishing
- ½ cup Green onion, sliced thinly

For peanut sauce:

- 1 tbsp. Rice Vinegar
- 2 tbsp. Hot Water
- ¼ cup Peanut Butter, natural
- 1/8 tsp. Sesame Oil, toasted

- 1 tbsp. Soy Sauce
- 1 tbsp. Agave Nectar

Direction:

1. To make this easy salad, you first need to heat water in a large pot over medium heat.
2. Once it starts boiling, stir in the broccoli and cook for half a minute.
3. After that, transfer the cooked broccoli to a strainer and place in a bowl of cold water.
4. Drain the broccoli and put in a large mixing bowl.
5. Add all the remaining salad ingredients to the bowl and toss well.
6. Now, make the peanut sauce by mixing all the ingredients needed to make the dressing in a bowl with a whisk. Set it aside.
7. Finally, spoon in the dressing and garnish it with the sesame seeds.

Nutrition:

543 Calories

36g Protein

85g Carbohydrates

33. Arugula Green Beans Salad

Preparation Time: 10 minutes

Cooking Time: 25 minutes

Serving: 8

Ingredients:

For salad:

- 2 handful of Arugula
- 4 tbsp. Capers
- 15 oz. Lentils, cooked
- 15 oz. Green Kidney Beans

For dressing:

- 1 tbsp. Balsamic Vinegar
- 1 tbsp. Tamari
- 2 tbsp. Peanut Butter
- 1 tbsp. Caper Brine
- 1 tbsp. Tahini
- 2 tbsp. Hot Sauce

Direction:

1. Begin by placing all the ingredients needed to make the dressing in a medium bowl and whisk it well until combined.
2. After that, combine the arugula, capers, kidney beans, and lentils in a large bowl. Pour the dressing over it.
3. Serve and enjoy.

Nutrition:

543 Calories

36g Protein

85g Carbohydrates

34. Black Bean Lentil Salad

Preparation Time: 10 minutes

Cooking Time: 20 minutes

Serving: 5

Ingredients:

- 1 Red Bell Pepper, diced
- 1 Cucumber, diced
- ½ of 1 Red Onion, small & diced
- 2/3 cup Cilantro
- 1 cup Green Lentils
- 2 Roma Tomatoes, diced
- 15 oz. Black Beans

For dressing:

- ½ tsp. Oregano
- Juice of 1 Lime
- 1/8 tsp. Salt
- 2 tbsp. Olive Oil
- 1 tsp. Cumin
- 1 tsp. Dijon Mustard
- 2 Garlic cloves

Direction:

1. To begin with, cook the lentils in a large pan over a medium heat following the manufacturer's instructions. Tip: The lentils should be cooked to firm but not mushy.
2. In the meantime, mix all the ingredients needed to make the dressing.
3. After that, combine the beans with the bell pepper, red onion cilantro, and cucumber. Spoon on the dressing.
4. Toss well and serve immediately.

Nutrition:

285 Calories

15g Protein

41g Carbohydrates

35. Quinoa Chickpeas Avocado Salad

Preparation Time: 10 minutes

Cooking Time: 20 minutes

Serving: 4

Ingredients:

- 1 Avocado
- 1 ½ tbsp. Tahini
- 30 Cherry Tomatoes, sliced
- 4 ½ cups Chickpeas, cooked
- ¼ tsp. Salt
- ½ of 1 Red Onion
- 1/3 cup Water
- 2 tbsp. Lemon Juice
- Pepper, as needed
- 1 ½ tsp. Dijon Mustard
- ½ cup Cilantro, packed

Direction:

1. To make this healthy salad, you first need to cook the quinoa by following the instructions given on the packet.
2. Next, take 1/3 rd. of the chickpeas and place in a high-speed blender along with the water, lemon juice, pepper, Dijon mustard, and salt.
3. Blend for a minute or until you get a creamy consistency.
4. Now, toss the cooked quinoa, cherry tomatoes, red onion, avocado, and cilantro into a large mixing bowl.
5. Drizzle the dressing over it and serve immediately.

Nutrition:

604 Calories

25g Protein

90g Carbohydrates

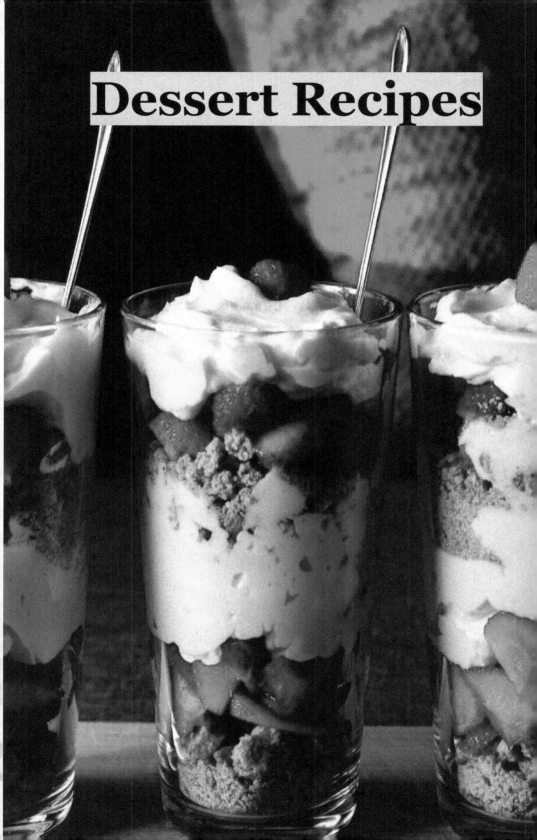

Dessert Recipes

36. Vegan Vanilla Ice Cream

Preparation Time: 15 minutes

Cooking Time: 45 minutes

Serving: 3

Ingredients:

- 3 vanilla pods
- 1 ½ tsp. vanilla bean paste
- 400 ml soymilk
- 600 grams light coconut milk
- 200 grams agave syrup

Directions:

1. Begin by slicing the vanilla pods and removing the seeds. Place the seeds in a big mixing bowl and toss out the pods. Next, add the rest of the ingredients, and position the ingredients into an ice cream maker. Churn the ice cream for forty-five minutes. Next, place the mixture into a freezer container, and allow the ice cream to freeze for three hours. Serve, and enjoy!

Nutrition

115 Calories

3g Fat

12g Protein

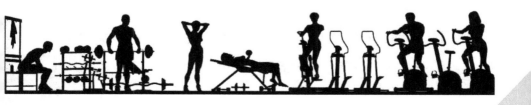

37. Watermelon Lollies

Preparation Time: 15 minutes

Cooking Time: 35 minutes

Servings: 5

Ingredients:

- ½ cup watermelon, cubed
- 2 tablespoons lemon juice, freshly squeezed
- ½ cup water
- 1 tablespoon stevia

Directions:

1. In a food processor, put cubed watermelon. Process until smooth. Divide an equal amount of the mixture into an ice pop container. Place inside the freezer for 1 hour.
2. Meanwhile, in a small bowl, put together lemon juice, water, and stevia. Mix well. Pour over frozen watermelon lollies. Add in pop sticks. Freeze for another hour.
3. Pry out watermelon lollies. Serve.

Nutrition

114 Calories

8g Fat

12g Protein

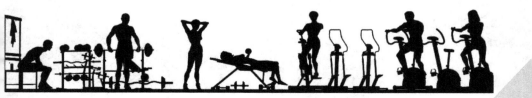

38. Lemon Bars

Preparation Time: 15 minutes

Cooking Time: 25 minutes

Servings: 5

Ingredients:

- 3/4 cup melted butter
- 3/4 cup almond flour
- 1 1/2 cups boiling water
- 2/3 cup lemon gelatin mix, no sugar added
- 3 Tbsp freshly squeezed lemon juice
- 12 oz cream cheese

Directions:

1. Set the oven to 350 degrees F.
2. Combine the melted butter and flour together in a bowl, then pour the mixture into a baking pan, pressing down to create a crust.
3. Bake for 10 minutes then set on a cooling rack. Cool completely before use.

4. In a large mixing bowl, mix the gelatin and boiling water. Stir until the gelatin completely dissolves.
5. Stir in the lemon juice and cream cheese, mixing well.
6. Pour the mixture on top of the crust, then place in the refrigerator and chill overnight, or for 3 hours at least.

Nutrition

119Calories

6g Fat

8g Protein

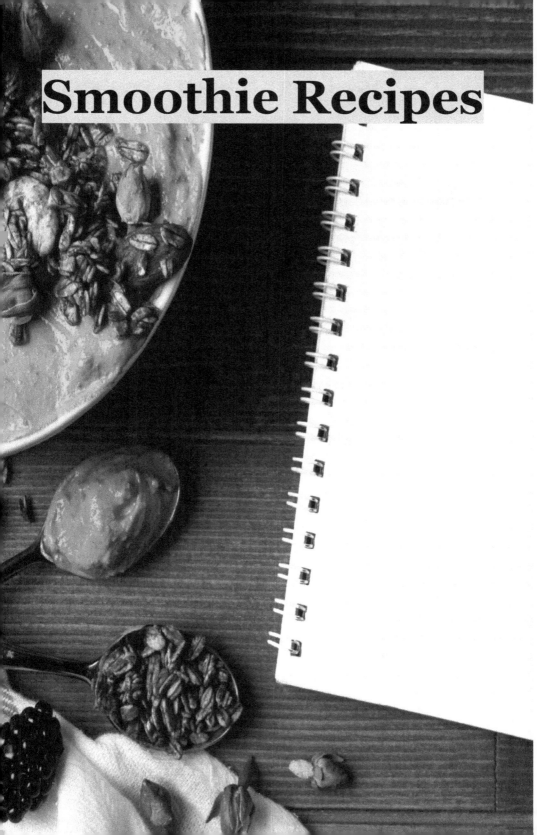

Smoothie Recipes

39. Tangy Spiced Cranberry Drink

Preparation Time: 10 minutes

Cooking Time: 3 hours

Servings: 14

Ingredients:

- 1 1/2 cups of coconut sugar
- 12 whole cloves
- 2 fluid ounce of lemon juice
- 6 fluid ounce of orange juice
- 32 fluid ounces of cranberry juice
- 8 cups of hot water
- 1/2 cup of Red-Hot candies

Directions:

1. Pour the water into a 6-quarts slow cooker along with the cranberry juice, orange juice, and the lemon juice.
2. Stir the sugar properly.

3. Wrap the whole cloves in a cheese cloth, tie its corners with strings, and immerse it in the liquid present inside the slow cooker.
4. Add the red-hot candies to the slow cooker and cover it with the lid.
5. Then plug in the slow cooker then cook on low heat until it is heated thoroughly.
6. When done, discard the cheesecloth bag and serve.

Nutrition:

89 Calories

27g Carbohydrates

3g Protein

40. Warm Pomegranate Punch

Preparation Time: 15 minutes

Cooking Time: 3 hours

Servings: 10

Ingredients:

- 3 cinnamon sticks
- 12 whole cloves
- 1/2 cup of coconut sugar
- 1/3 cup of lemon juice
- 32 fluid ounce of pomegranate juice
- 32 fluid ounce of apple juice, unsweetened
- 16 fluid ounces of brewed tea

Directions:

1. Using a 4-quart slow cooker, pour the lemon juice, pomegranate, juice apple juice, tea, and then sugar.
2. Wrap the whole cloves and cinnamon stick in a cheese cloth, tie its corners with a string, and immerse it in the liquid present in the slow cooker.

3. Then cover it with the lid, plug in the slow cooker and let it cook at the low heat setting for 3 hours or until it is heated thoroughly.
4. When done, discard the cheesecloth bag and serve it hot or cold.

Nutrition:

253 Calories

58g Carbohydrates

7g Protein

Conclusion

Thanks for making it to the end of this guide.

A plant-based diet provides a simple, effective way to cut processed foods from your diet. As well as being in my mind, healthier than animal-based products, plant-based products are cheaper. Plus, as long as you eat the appropriate variety, it's likely that a plant-based diet is nutritionally sufficient. Moreover, a plant-based diet is more ethical than an animal-based diet. The grain fed to livestock could be feeding humans. Animals have to endure a lifetime on factory farms. Plants however don't endure anything. They grow and then die. They don't produce waste or pollution. They don't consume any resources. It should be pretty clear that a plant-based diet is, environmentally speaking, the way we should eat. Still, individuals often assume a plant-based diet isn't complete enough unless you add in the meat.

It's easy to assume that humans aren't likely to thrive without adding meat. But it turns out that we're doing just fine. For example, many of the wealthiest countries have diets that are heavily plant-based—yet they also have among the lowest rates of diet-related diseases. Unlike plants, animals are used for meat, milk, and eggs. But those products only provide a small fraction of the essential nutrients for optimal health. The majority of protein a healthy person need comes from plants. Animal protein is no different in this regard. Simply by switching to a plant-based diet you will soon discover that you can still get enough protein—even if you're a meat-eater. However, plant protein is far superior to animal protein. The proteins in animal products increase the risk of breast cancer, prostate cancer, cardiovascular disease, diabetes, and other illnesses.

Plant protein, on the other hand, reduces the risks of those diseases. The protein in plants is high in fiber and low in saturated fat. A plant-based diet is also rich in antioxidants—particularly vitamin C. Plant-based antioxidants actually reduce cholesterol levels. They also help the body deal with heat stress and provide support for the immune system.

In a nutshell, a plant-based diet is far more fulfilling than animal-based products. Although a plant-based diet may seem more expensive than animal-based products, this isn't the case. The meat, dairy and egg industries are heavily subsidized with public money. This makes their products cheap. Meanwhile, plants are often priced according to how much water and fuel they require. As a result, many of the world's population pays more for animal products than they would for plants. A plant-based diet is healthier and more environmentally sound—as well as more ethical. What's not to love?

Humans have long enjoyed eating plant-based food. Even the earliest hunter-gatherers ate increasingly fewer plants as they started hunting more and more animals. Over time, plant-based food became rarer and rarer among the world's meat-eating communities. As a result, plant-based food is now considered a luxury in much of the world. People may not consider it luxurious, but animals certainly do. They don't actually care what they eat. They don't choose to be eaten any more than we choose to eat plants. They don't even know our language. But needless to say, we wouldn't employ, slaughter and eat animals like we currently do if we tried to think like them.

If we took an animal's perspective, the way we raise animals for food would be repulsive. Despite the fact that this is what animals think—and that the way we treat them is painful and unfair, we still believe we have the right to consume them and use them for material gain. If we were to look at the situation from an animal's perspective, the only conclusion to be drawn is that we have no right to exploit them for our own consumption—let alone the consumption of their own families. Although some individuals have now embraced a plant-based diet, the vast majority of people still consume an animal-based diet.

CPSIA information can be obtained
at www.ICGtesting.com
Printed in the USA
BVHW051355270421
605941BV00002B/91

9 781802 450200